Bedtime Stories for Adults

9 Relaxing Sleep Stories for Everyday Guided Meditation, Mindfulness for Beginners, Self Hypnosis, Anxiety & Spiritual Brain Healing

Written By

Lucy Holden

Lucy Holden

© Copyright 2019 Lucy Holden all rights reserved.

The content contained within this book may not be reproduced, duplicated or transmitted without direct written permission from the author or the publisher.

Under no circumstances will any blame or legal responsibility be held against the publisher, or author, for any damages, reparation, or monetary loss due to the information contained within this book. Either directly or indirectly.

Legal Notice:

This book is copyright protected. This book is only for personal use. You cannot amend, distribute, sell, use, quote or paraphrase any part, or the content within this book, without the consent of the author or publisher.

Disclaimer Notice:

Please note the information contained within this document is for educational and entertainment purposes only. All effort has been executed to present accurate, up to date, and reliable, complete information. No warranties of any kind are declared or implied. Readers acknowledge that the author is not engaging in the rendering of legal, financial, medical or professional advice. The content within this book has been derived from various sources. Please consult a licensed professional before attempting any techniques outlined in this book.

By reading this document, the reader agrees that under no circumstances is the author responsible for any losses, direct or indirect, which are incurred as a result of the use of information contained within this document, including, but not limited to, — errors, omissions, or inaccuracies.

Lucy Holden

Contents

The Secret Cabin   5

The Genius 13

The Hot Air Balloon   19

The Magic Library   26

The Enchanted World   33

The Tranquil Submarine   39

The Dream Life 46

The Ocean's Song   52

The Changing Seasons   59

The Secret Cabin

You have just left your car in the safe lot behind you. You walk upon the woods from the graveled lot, as you make your way onto the path you stop to admire the beauty. You close your eyes as you look up through the autumn leaves. Feeling the sunlight warm your face and smelling the crispness of the turned leaves. As the sun light dances behind your eyelids you feel yourself calm and relax, ready to journey through this forest of warm sunshine and mellow color. Opening your eyes as you lower you head back you take in all the richness around you. Many of the trees full with vibrant colors, some are evergreen, and some are showing their branches as their shaken off the old and are ready to embrace the new. You haven't explored this forest before, but you are going to meet a friend in cozy cabin that is deep in the forest.

This small get away and escape from our technical world is exactly what you need. Taking a deep breath, you start to wander down the well-worn foot path. The path welcoming you as it has many strangers in the past. As you walk the leaves giving a slight, satisfying crunch as your comfy hiking shoes cradle your feet.   The once lush forest is in preparation for the upcoming winter.   Just like your body settles in for the rest, it must prepare. As you feel your body settling in to the autumnal shifts you notice the squirrels scurrying about, collecting their supply for their own long rest. The birds have mostly headed south and the only noise you can hear is the slight rustle of the leaves as a crisp wind blows through.

As you keep exploring into the woods, you come up on a large pine tree. You stop to briefly admire it, and you are amazed by the sheer size of it. This is the biggest tree you have ever seen. You cannot even see the very top, just lush and thick, deep green branches all the way to the top. You wonder how long this tree has been here. The things it must have been around to experience. Perhaps this tree was only a tiny sapling when your great, great ancestors were establishing the family that would eventually lead to you. Of all the cosmic events and paths of mother nature, one has led to you. Just like the many stages in your life they all have a beginning and an ending.   Nature is pleasantly predictable as

Bedtime Stories for Adults

all things follow a natural order, the sun rises, the sun sets, and a new day comes. You must rest in between to have a long, healthy life. This seed was planted. With nourishment it began to grow. Despite all odds, life continues. Saplings are able to grow into gigantic pine trees. You feel that slight breeze as it blows through and ruffles your hair, reminding you that you need to reach the cabin. You continue on the footpath... further from the city, closer to the still calmness of forest. The sounds of the city and busy roads are far behind you now. A distant memory as your body adjusts to the new sounds in the forest. Your body openly accepts the welcoming relaxation that the world is providing.

Your eyes relax with the warm colors surrounding you, the deep amber, the golden yellows, and the harvest orange of the leaves. You meander through the wooded land and you notice a new sound. A pleasant sound of the faintest trickle of a babbling brook. As you travel closer to the brook you can see the stream flowing smooth and calm, causing the smallest of waterfalls as the water caresses the round rocks. There is a striking green moss around the stream causing an ethereal appearance to this mystical place. The stream, clear and meandering feels fresh, like it could wash away all your troubles just by being near it. Let the stream carry away any thoughts that are hindering you. Toss them into the stream and they can be washed away for another time. You watch your troubles slip away on the surface of the stream and you start to walk along beside the water.

As the stream wraps around the path you see a small wooden bridge arcing over the pathway. Weather worn but sturdy the bridge gives a little sigh as you walk across it. Holding on to the handrail you can feel the warmth from the sun radiating through your body. Though all this land is new for you, it oddly feels like coming home. Like the surrounding warmth you feel around you is familiar. It welcomes you with open arms and you wonder how much longer until you'll reach the cabin, how wonderful will it be? A little up ahead you can see a split in the path, as you get closer you can read the hand carved sign pointing to the right. Nightingale cabin is very close. Only a short distance to travel and you'll be ready for your vacation of peace and relaxation. The dense forest starts to give way to bigger rocks, hinting that you have explored yourself further to edge of the mountain. To the left you can see as the vegetation has thinned out to make way for mountain cliffs, you will explore those later. For now, you just want to settle in.

Your pack starts to feel heavy on you. As if it has been weighing your body down with every step. Your legs long to rest, but you know there is not much further to go. Up ahead on the horizon you see the cabin. The green tin roof stands out against the autumn colors surrounding it. The welcoming warm woods and white trim make this cabin appear to be cozier than its grand scale depicts. The round logs only giving way to grand white framed windows. Your tiredness turns into relief as you walk up the three short stairs to the welcoming door. Seeing a note on the door you read that your friend has went out briefly but will return in a while. In the meantime, you are instructed to make yourself at home. You turn the knob and open the door, as you move through the threshold there is one sight that captivates you.

Lucy Holden

The large sightseeing windows provide a picturesque mountain overlook as you can now see the cabin is perched near a cliff. The colorful trees, spotted with occasional evergreens is breath taking. You focus on your breathing as you look among the trees, breathing in, then slowly releasing that breath. How many different colors can you see? Breathing in you count 1, 2, 3. Breathing out you count more. Do this until you've discovered all the colors there are to be seen in this beautiful forest that surrounds you. This welcoming home away from home.

You take off your pack and notice the kitchenette is to the left, the rooms off to the right, but directly ahead of you in front of the welcoming windows is a great room. You set your pack on the table by the entrance for now. You'll settle in your things later. Now it is time to rest your body. The great room has a fire place with wood and kindling ready to go, you notice the slight chill in the air so you decide starting a small fire is a good idea. You take the small logs from the top of the pile, along with some kindling, and place them into the fire place. You notice the matches on a coffee table behind you and you use them to light this fire. As the small fire blossoms to life with a small roar and crackles you can feel the heat drifting off it. Feeling the warmth makes you realize there is a slight coldness that has seeped in from walking through the autumn forest. You look around the great room. Seeing the warm colors in the cabin reflecting those that are all around you in the woods.

There is an inviting brown leather sofa in the center of the room, with a deep red throw. You lie down on the sofa and sink down further into the comfort, pulling the throw around you and banishing all cold from your body. The warmth surrounding you as you hear the slight crackle of the fire. A light rain has started out side and you can hear the pitter patter on the green tin roof as you see the cold rain falling outside you are grateful to be inside. Warm and cozy, with softness snuggled all around you. As you close your eyes again you can feel the warm colors comforting your senses. The cabin is quiet, your mind is relaxed, your body finally relaxes fully. Letting your arms down to your fingers drift off to sleep. Your neck and all down your spine, sinks into the sofa, relaxing on the most comfortable surface. Your legs all the way down to your toes sink further down off to sleep. You mind drifts of to relax with the rest of your body. Let it relax, there is nothing holding you back. Your vacation starts now, your only job is to let everything slip away as your mind embraces the nothingness that is complete peace.

The Genius

Tonight, we are going to witness the power of the human mind. An extraordinary existence that lies within you and the power within it has so much untapped potential. We are going to tap into that genius potential to give you the most relaxing and serene peace that your body and mind have ever experienced. First, you must clear your mind. Let's do this with an organizational approach. Imagine a room; it can be stark white, it can be an ordinary office; maybe it's a storage room, or an extraterrestrial room that is dark with sleek modern touches. This room will be your way to file and organize your thoughts, putting them away for the night.

Let us start collecting those thoughts, by exploring your thought super highway and gathering everything we can find. Collect the thoughts however you need; if they are organized maybe you can set up a road block. Position yourself to slow, then halt the thoughts, processing which way they need to go. Compressing the thoughts into tiny manageable pieces. Maybe your thoughts are scattered, you can lay a net or a trap, and gather them all up at once? Then take each thought, figure out what it is, assign it to a file. As all the thoughts ramble and bounce around in your mind, stop them and gather them into a pile. Maybe some thoughts are linked together, place them within the same file or box; however big you need that storage bin or containment system to be. Your stack is growing higher and higher as all the thoughts from the day leave your thought highway and go into your manageable file system.

Once you have a hefty pile, you lift it up. The weight feeling like a burden and weighing you down, you take the thoughts to your organizational room. Let's begin filing away these thoughts. Stacking them, filing them, whatever you need to do to clean up your mind space. Making things nice, tidy, and neat. Take your time, go through every thought, making sure it is tucked away, not going to fall off and ramble its way back onto the thought highway.   If you feel any loose thoughts escaping, making their way back onto the thought highway, let it go, don't fight it. Finish putting away what you have now, these thoughts are ready to be put to rest. Once everything is put in its place, go back to the highway for a last sweep. Any errant thoughts can be grabbed up now. Catch those thoughts and take them back to the organization room. Are all your thoughts tucked away? If yes, your mind is blank and ready to explore? If no, take a moment and keep collecting and storing until you're ready to move on.

You leave the organization room behind you now. You travel through your mind, we're going to tap into the

Bedtime Stories for Adults

parts you do not use often enough. You can visualize your brain, the parts you use often are alive and electric. As you pass these parts by, allow them to calm down. Let them rest, they have done enough for today, we don't need them for what we are going to do. You pass by the central part, the one that controls your breathing, you heart rate, gently caress it. Let it know it can relax too, it can slow down. Feel your breathing calm, your heart rate a soft cadence; the reassurance that life is within you and will continue to be so in the morning. As you feel your mind relaxing you continue to travel through. Passing the parts, you do not use enough, seeing them with their soft warm glow, welcoming you to tap into them. Once you have located the untapped potential, touch it. Reach up your arms and stretch them long. Stretch your torso and back, twist to reach it. Make your legs long all the way to your toes. Now you feel it, you're touching this dull area and a warm sensation is starting to come alive and you can feel it washing over you. It starts to warm up and emit a little happy glow that travels all through your body. Your muscles start to relax as the warmness caress it, your mind feels pleasant, bubbling and cloudy, until it sinks into the warm, soft light, then you can see a vivid green field all around you.

The sky is blue, the tall grass, soft and green. Your entire body feels warm and relaxed. Let's see if this is the true potential of your mind with a little test. Imagine yellow dandelions growing all over the field. Big ones, small ones. Count them as you add the yellow dandelions, until you can't count. There's too many, millions and millions of yellow flowers surrounding you with happiness and joy. This is the power of your mind, if your mind isn't cooperating then you're not ready for this area. Don't give up, go back, explore your brain, find another untapped area and keep trying. You will find one that will let you explore. Once you're in a warm area and you see the field that you can control, you are there. Now that we are all there let's practice this new and pleasing sensation of control, turn the dandelions into to their fluffy white flowers, ready to release their seeds into the world. All around you, in a field full of white fluffy dandelions. Pick one up. Take a deep breath in, then blow it out slowly. Watching the seeds spiral from the flower into the air. As the seeds float back to the earth, steady yourself. This is just a very small power that rests inside you, it can do so much more. Take another deep breath in as you pick another dandelion. Exhale as you blow those seeds and come to terms with the fact you are a genius. You are capable of anything you set your mind to. Rest and relaxation can help you tap into that genius.

You command your mind and body. Right now, you command them to relax. Your entire body is soft, relaxed, and pliable. Your mind is warm, enriched, and welcoming to the thoughts of your tapped genius

Bedtime Stories for Adults

potential. You can go anywhere in the world right now, without leaving this state of relaxation. Where do you want to go? Picture that place; is it an ocean shore, a busy city, a small village, or a place you know well? What does it smell like? What can you hear? What can you see? How does it make you feel? Take a moment and enjoy this place, explore the sensations. Is it everything you hoped it would be?

This is your mind allowing you to experience the most wonderful sensations whenever you want it to. This power is incredible. You want to be on a beach in Greece, done. You want to be in the mountains in Asia, done. You want to be anywhere in space or time, you can do that. You are a wonderful, amazing creature, with limitless abilities as you bring yourself into ultimate relaxation at the same time. Would you like to see what else your mind is capable of?

Picture the tallest building in the world. Now get to the top of it. How does your mind get you there? Do you instantly appear on the top of the building? Do you walk up to the building, enter, and take an elevator? Do you start the arduous task of climbing the stairs? Do you gear up and climb the side of the building? Or maybe you come from above, using a parachute as you fall from a plane to land on top of the tallest building in the world. So many possibilities can spring from one simple suggestion. If you can get to the top of this building, then you can do anything. Take your time, or get it done quickly. It doesn't matter, because all the potential to do it, is inside your mind.

Can you understand now how beautiful and creative your mind is? Your mind can grow and continue to astound you every day, if you let it. Listen to your mind, let it guide you... Let your mind connect with your heart, picture the direct link between the two. This connection will know what you want the most in this life. Do not stop it, do not slow it down. Let it carry you away, showing you your hopes and dreams and how you can achieve them. Stay in this state of relaxation, do not let the errant thoughts break out of their storage room. They are locked away, stored nice and neatly for tomorrow. Tonight, is not about any of those thoughts, quickly lock that door, then forget it. It is about you, who you are, what you want, and how you are going to get it.

Everything becomes clear and easy to manage. Just like organizing your thoughts, your mind can control and process anything you bring its way. Let it take over, just as it took you into this deep relaxation. Once you are in total control of your mind, then you can shut it down and go to sleep. Enjoy your peaceful rest, and I look forward to seeing your genius potential in the world.

The Hot Air Balloon

You feel the excitement and nervousness in your restless body as you approach the gigantic balloon. Climbing into the wicker basket, you feel your heart flutter and your stomach do a small flip.   You can smell the propane and hear the burning flame ready to power this balloon into the air. Holding onto the edge of the basket you wait for your secure ascent into the air. Feeling the smooth wood beneath your hand, the drift of the slightest amount of heat from the balloon, the distant smell of a salty ocean. As the basket starts to rise you feel how tense and achy your muscles are. You concentrate on grounding yourself as your body is being lifted to unknown heights.

Digging your toes down into the floor of the basket. Feeling your strong, sturdy ankles supporting you letting you know they won't waver, they will keep you steady. Your legs feel alive as the muscles reflectively tense and relax as you ground yourself. As you rise even higher you feel a shift in your body. The fear of the flight is leaving you, and instead you feel an uplifting grace and peaceful presence. Your body doesn't feel as heavy as it did moments ago. The almost weightlessness you experience settles you. As you look around at the beautiful scenery you continue to stabilize your body. Relaxing your aching back, allowing the curves to blend into themselves. Your stomach settling down as you focus your thoughts into your breathing. Breathing in and expanding your lungs, delivering oxygen to your body. Breathing out, allowing your muscles to relax and await their next oxygen delivery. As you breath in and out slowly, you are able to relax your shoulders, neck, and finally your mind.

As you continue relaxing and breathing, you are able to focus on the land growing smaller beneath you. Like the troubles you leave behind when you sleep. The balloon drifts peacefully, you can see the ocean now. The water deep blue, the beach over-crowded as people are eager to find the blissful relaxation that you're already able to experience. The red and white umbrellas line the crowded beach, people lying on their towels on the warm sand. You're above the beach now and people point and you can hear them hoot and holler as you soar above. Hearing the ocean lull beneath the sound of the crowd. You wave hello with a warm smile, thankful you can easily slip away from this crowded area and into your own cocoon of happiness and warmth. The balloon drifts further from the crowd and noises. The ocean shrinking and becoming distant. You can no longer smell or hear the bustle that was on the ocean shore. Now, your mind is welcoming the quiet uninhabited lands you are approaching. You nose is eager for the clean crisp scents of the fields beneath you.

Bedtime Stories for Adults

Seeing many colors of wild flowers blur together as you soar above. Like a bird in a lengthy flight for winter, you take in all your surroundings. Relaxing, breathing, just being. Traveling away for your long, peaceful rest. Stepping away from the cold harshness that can sometimes be reality, and traveling to the warm, sunny peace deep inside your mind. Below you see a laundry line and a small farm house; seeing the clothing dance on the line as you gently pass by, as if now they are waving to you as you waved to the beach goers. The land turns from flat and uninhabited to small rolling hills with the occasional house.

You see the town grow as you travel towards the center, more roads, more houses, and more businesses. Like the path of your life; you start out fresh, not knowing many things, being able to see and know everything around you like the small farm house. As you age, the roads you travel become familiar, but longer, more complicated, twists and turns, connecting to other roads. The houses keep popping up as you meet new people. The businesses are opportunities that you may latch onto or let them pass by; whichever is right for you at that time in your life. The connections throughout this town or city, working like your mind often does. Growing together, supporting a singular body.

Lucy Holden

You pass over neighborhoods, seeing the quiet towns below. Friendly neighbors having cookouts and children playing kick ball together. The towns pass by so quickly and it reminds you of how quick time can seem to pass. Your mind tries to distract you, remind you of the things you need to accomplish. The things you need to worry about. It's time to quiet those thoughts. You are creating your own wind as you soar through the sky, whisper your concerns to the wind. Let them travel through the air, fall to the ground. You can pick them up at another time. Whisper the thoughts of what you need to do tomorrow. Whisper the thoughts of what you should be worrying about. Whisper anything that is on your mind. Watch the words leave your mouth, drift through your wind, fall to the ground. The words jumbling together as they spiral to the ground. Falling and falling until you can no longer see them. Those thoughts are gone now; you have freed your mind and have total control over your body.

Breathing in allowing your body to soak in the peace with a clear mind. Breathing out feeling your body sigh with relief. The hot air balloon is now traveling over the forest. The tops of the trees are green and lush. You feel like a cloud floating above the trees. The coverage dense in some areas, shielding you from the world below. While in other areas it thins out, allowing you to peek at the wonder mother nature has set before you.

Bedtime Stories for Adults

A group of birds' flocks beside you, you can hear them calling out to each other at the curiosity you are presenting to them in this huge balloon. How odd it must be for them. You look up and are again amazed at how a little bit of heat and this huge material are allowing you to soar with birds. The rainbow color panels seem to glow as the sun shines down through them. The red panel making you think of love and warmth. The orange panel reminding you of tropical colors on an island, the flowers, the clothes, the fruits, and the peaceful setting sun. The yellow panel reminding you of pure happiness and joy; like a full warm sun, or the tart bite of a lemon. The green panel showing the reflection of life; of mother nature as it surrounds you...the green of the trees, the grass, the fields below. The blue panel, reflecting on the open clear skies. Open like your mind, absorbing the welcoming warmth of the other colors. The purple panel, reflecting its vibrant color that can be rarer than the others and is often a sign of nobility. Reflecting the rare peace and calm of complete bliss, reflecting this journey in this hot air balloon.

The forest is thinning out and you can see a beach in the distance. As you approach it you find yourself approaching a barely sandy and more rocky shore, the water angrily lapping at the shoreline. While not friendly for a relaxing day at the beach, the sounds of the crashing waves reflect that of your beating heart. It's as if you can feel those waves beating against the rocks from deep within your soul. You feel the blood pumping through your body, then beating through your heart. The waves rolling in and out like your breath. Working together to create a beautiful rhythm that is essential for your life. The sounds of the ocean start to drift off until you only feel your heart, mirroring what you know the ocean is doing even in your absence.

You approach an open field, you know your journey must be near its end. As the balloon starts to descend, you feel yourself falling slightly more horizontal. Peacefully drifting into the proper place of relaxation. Your body shifts, finding the most comforting position as you feel the weight returning to your body. The heaviness weighing your body down until it feels impossible to do nothing but let it pull you down. Relax into the weight. Feel your body sinking into the warmth of the descent. Allow your tired legs to rest, pulling the rest of your body down with them. Breath in and out slowly as you drift down into peace, lying your head back and feeling gravity welcome you home. The warmth of the balloon envelopes you as you caress the ground. The balloon is at rest. Lie here as long as you like. Rest, breath in the field around you. What does this field look like up closely? Is it fragrant flowers? Warm and mellow wheat? Close your eyes and rest for a moment. Allow your body to sink in and enjoy this complete relaxation this trip has brought you. Reflect on the sights that you have seen, only one thing stirs you from your revelry... The pilot asks you, "Do you want to go up again?"

Lucy Holden

The Magic Library

Tonight, you are going to visit a special library. You have been told that this particular library is magical, people leave here in an elevated state that simply can't be explained. For this reason, you are going to experience the magic for yourself. You notice this small town is very homey as you walk down the sidewalk. There is a small grocery store on the left, already closed, though the night still feels early. Beside it are a few office buildings, a lawyer, a real estate agent, a postal building. With almost every business sleeping, you wonder why the library never closes? Who hires a night shift for a library, when even places like the grocery store are closing at sun down? What an odd town this is seeming to be...

As you walk down the nearly deserted streets, enjoying the picturesque small town, you watch the lamp posts come to life. As they light up one by one, you realize they're not light bulbs, but old-timey gas light posts. The warm glow emits a soft light and feels like you're transporting to an older time. You check the time on your cell phone, but mainly just to make sure it is still working. Shaking off the odd sensation and putting your phone away for good, you continue on to the library. You come to the town square and know you are getting close to the famed library.

Bedtime Stories for Adults

There is a small movie theater to your right, only showing one picture. You remember the film from weeks ago, this poor town must be the very last to receive new films. At least this theater is open, unlike the many other businesses, with its lights helping illuminate the poorly lit sidewalk. A few other boutiques are around the square, with a large aged limestone building in the center. You realize this building in the center is the town courthouse from the engraving on the side of the building. Instead of going all the way around the square, you walk straight through to the road behind it.

The stars are flickering to life above you. You stand on the sidewalk and admire how bright the night sky can be when the lights from the town don't reach very high. Seeing constellations, you can't name, and you feel as though you can see every star there is. A bright blue one, one that's slightly red, noticing the planets with your bare eye and wondering the works of Galileo.   There are some that are so bright, some that flicker, some that aren't as bright, as if to say they're tired. A slight chill stops your revelry as you remember you are here to visit this library, not stare at the stars all night. You continue your walk and you come upon a very old building in the distance. From what you have heard, this must be the library.

Lucy Holden

As you get closer you notice the details of this magnificent place. The architecture reflecting the court house that was in the center of the square. The pristine white of the limestone is long gone, as if to make way for the delicate aging process. A large antique clock is centered on the face of the library, but the time is accurate. Peeling your eyes away from the building to admire the well-kept grounds. The green space is large and has many cozy nooks to cuddle in while you read. There is a small pond on the side, with benches and cattails. You won't go explore it yet, but you know there must be goldfish and probably even ducks that come visit. There are large trees that are perfect to lean against and have shade while you're reading on a warm summer day. The willows towards the back of the ground must be like a world of their own to lie beneath their umbrella and experience a small bubble of peace around you.

You're eager to go inside and you've finally reached the stairs, they are nearly as wide as the face of the building and only 5 tall. As you walk up them, you hope you're not disappointed. A library is a place to rent books, yes, this one is different because it never closes, but it still has the same purpose. There are benches along the front of the library for those that can't wait to take their books home. The gas lamps help illuminate, but it's too poorly lit for readers at night. Taking a deep breath of fresh air, you grab on the handle of the wooden door and pull.

Bedtime Stories for Adults

Walking through the threshold you feel a stillness in the air, while it is typical for libraries, this is different. The air feels electric, like it is being forced to stay still. The marble floors shine, the deep wooden shelves contrast against them. A large circular desk in the center beholds one small lady that gives you a kind smile. Towards the back left there are signs pointing to the kid's area. Stairs that lead down to the 'Local History and Genealogy' area. Turning your attention to the right, you see the various sections. You start to walk down each. Smelling the crisp book scent, as you walk up and down each isle. You touch the spines of a few books, caressing the different types of materials. The leather-bound ones are rare, but feel the smoothest as you run your fingers across them. The hardbacks feeling rough compared to the softness of the others.

You admire the hard work that went into organizing these books. If you could fix your own life problems by applying a similar method, how simple could your life become? Try that now, what problems are most troublesome? Once you have your thoughts, visualize writing them down. Following the curve of your pen in your mind as you write the troubles, turning them into just words. Place that paper inside your mind book. What does your mind book look like? Is it leather-bound and sturdy? Is it hard-back and rough to the touch? Is it a large book or a small book? Are the pages thick and sturdy, or thin and delicate? Turn the page, write any other thoughts down so you can save them for later. Anything that is on your mind, write it down, follow the pen, taking thoughts and making them only words. Once your mind book contains anything clouding your mind, snap it closed. Place it on to the shelf and let's explore. Free from thoughts, opening our senses, ready to relax and enjoy the magic you've been feeling in the air.

Walking into your favorite section of books you feel a warm happiness wash over you. Ready to experience the magic, your hands eagerly search for the book that is calling out to your soul. As you search, your arms begin to feel heavy and tired. You back and legs are becoming stiff, you pause for a moment to stretch. Reaching your arms up tall, twisting a little bit, side to side, stretching your toes down, then relaxing it all. As you touch the shelf again, your hand rests on the book. This is the book you would like to explore. You take the book from the self and carry it with you to the little alcove with a big comfy chair. You sit in the chair and move around until you sink into complete comfort.

There is no one around. It is just you, this book, and the most comfortable chair you've ever sat in. Your body sighs with relief as every muscle begins to relax. Take a moment, allowing every muscle time to just settle. The muscles between your toes, across the bottom, then the

Bedtime Stories for Adults

tops of your feet. From your ankles up to your knees, relaxing. Your bottom, your spine, your stomach; relax and enjoy the pleasant sensation of total relaxation. As you feel your body melding to the chair, your chest eases into a slow pattern, breathing in, then out. You feel the breath radiating warm, peaceful messages to your tired arms. Letting every muscle experience that breath as if comes down in between your fingers, then back up all the way to between your shoulders. Your shoulders relaxing, pulling down on the muscles in your neck. And then finally, up to your brain. Relaxation coaxing your brain, the synapses settling. Your entire body is warm, soft, relaxed. Now it is time to read your book.

You open the book and feel your eyes becoming heavy as you read the first few lines. The book feels heavy in your hand. Let the book drop on to your lap, rest your hands. Watch the words drift together, then close your eyes to let them rest. As you begin to drift, you hear a soothing voice read you your story. You lie your head back against the chair and feel yourself drifting peacefully as you enjoy your book. You learn about the characters in the book, what they look like, things they enjoy, their personality. As you listen to the book in your mind, you realize you have total control over everything. Every thought you may have becomes a part of the book. The narrator easily adapts your thoughts and continues with entertaining your resting mind. The story is now your

Lucy Holden

own, keep your mind and body relaxed and enjoy your time at the library.

The Enchanted World

Your head feels foggy as you try to remember where you are and how you came to be here, but there is nothing. As you peer up through half open eyes you see an astounding night sky, but it is very different from anything you have seen before. The sky is not black, but rather a deep purple with blue clouds. There is not one, but two moons. One is very similar to the one that you've seen your entire life, while the other is twice the size and glistens with silvery light off its smooth surface. The big moon reminds you of the time when you broke a thermometer and the silver liquid pools together, moving differently from other liquids. The stars are few and far between, some large, some small...but they are all a violet hue. Some are light purple, the softest violet. Some are dark, you can barely notice them except for their sparkle allowing them to be revealed.

You feel the ground beneath you, solid, but warm. As if the earth itself is a being, there to support you. The soft grass like a gentle wool blanket beneath you. You become more aware of your body ascertaining your well-being in this foreign place. Your body feels tired, heavy. You slowly rise to your feet, allowing your tired body to feel the gravity of this new place. When you stand, you want nothing more than to lie back down on the warm, satisfying earth...but you must know why you are here. And where is here?

As you look around you, you notice it is dark, but not total darkness. Some of the plants let off luminescent hues of blues, greens, and purples. As you take a step, the warm earth lets off a soft light, illuminating the pressure beneath your feet. It is as if it is saying it will help you light the way. You stare at your feet as the soft rings of blue and green emanate from your feet. You take another step, and watch the lights follow. This fantasy world is so remarkable, you feel as though you are inside a dream.

You walk by tall, whimsical flowers, as you reach out and touch them, they not only glow they let out small chimes of music. Their rosy hues stand out amongst the other colors and they smell so fragrant. Their petals soft like satin, glow the softest of pink on the inside, and a darker rose on the ends. You run your fingers through the flowers, listening to the tinkling chimes. Oddly playing with these strange flowers, you realize this place is even more strange. You attempt to look beyond this forest, but it seems the forest can go on for days and days. You can feel the hunger for survival starting to wake up inside you. Looking around you search for other signs of life; for rodents, insects, flying creatures, but you see nothing.

Bedtime Stories for Adults

It seems the only living things here are you, the plants, and the very earth itself.

The feeling of hopelessness and defeat come next. What is this place? Why are you here? How will you survive? What of your loved ones? You feel an odd sensation as a strange deep voice speaks inside your head. "Worry not, my child. Tell me your troubles, for that is why you are here." Startled at the intrusion you sink down and sit silently, but you are not scared. What damage can it do to share your troubles? So, tell the voice your problems. What has been bothering you? You can feel it listening to you, with a comforting ear. As you list off your sorrows, you can feel them leaving your body. Nothing but warmth filling your soul as the troubles slip away into the ear of this being. I'll give you a moment alone now, to let yourself rid your body of any negative or troublesome thoughts.

As you sit in silence and have finally banished all the negativity from your mind you hear the welcoming voice, "Now, I have taken away anything that weighs down heavily on your soul. All is well, you are safe. Your loved ones are safe. Your soul will be light and not weigh you down as you travel. Enjoy this journey, find the things you seek, and then you shall return home."

Your mind feels settled and quiet, you know the being is not in there anymore. You are alone, but comforted.

Lucy Holden

Your body does not feel heavy now, it feels so light. You jump to see how light you feel and you go a great distance in the air, but you're not scared as you float gently back down. Seeing the tops of the trees with their vines hanging down around them. Watching the pulsing luminescence waving hello as you pass them by. You softly land amazed there is no fear, only joy as you prepare to go again. You take a deep breath in as you launch yourself, this time fully aware of what you are doing. Stretching your muscles out, as your eyes eagerly take in the breath-taking landscape. Breathing out as you float back down to the ground. Breathing in again as you jump up, then slowly exhaling as you float back down.

Your legs are starting to feel tired, but there is something that has caught your eye and you must try to see it again. You jump up one last time, and yes, there it is, not far in the distance is a waterfall. It is very tall, and you want to go see it up close. Floating back down to earth you let your sensations adapt to the new weightlessness of your body. You start to head in the direction of the waterfall. You are enjoying the magical lights as you wander through the forest. Watching your feet dance a magical path as they light up the way. As you get closer you can hear the rushing water falling from its great height and your heart is filled with joy. It is as if all sadness that was ever in your heart or mind is banished. There is no room for anything but pure joy and happiness.

Bedtime Stories for Adults

Your face smiles, reflecting how the rest of your mind and body feel as you finally see the waterfall up close. It is at least 3 stories tall, but the water doesn't rush and push everything out of its way. It caresses the rocks, smoothing rough edges. Floating down into the pristine pool beneath it, much like your body floats in this magical place. Inside the pristine pool are tiny orbs of white light. You make your way close to the water's surface to inspect these curiosities. You dip your hands in and scoop up the tiny orb, as you bring it closer to your face to inspect, you see a tiny person that is letting off this orb of light. She reaches out to pop the bubble, shakes the water off, spreads out beautiful, tiny white wings and flies away.

You watch her tiny light growing dimmer and dimmer as she flies up until you can no longer see her. You sit beside the water and admire the other orbs in the water, that must be the same creature you just encountered. As you sit patiently, you see some of the orbs come to the surface; and just like the one you witnessed, they pop their bubbles and fly off. Afraid to speak and disturb this event, you only watch. The tiny light orbs rise, burst gracefully, then a tiny fairy takes her flight. As more and more rise to the surface and then take flight it is like the stars falling in reverse. More and more, they bubble up from deep down in the water, break the surface, shake themselves free, then rise.

Lucy Holden

You feel your body calling down to snuggle against the warm earth, so you indulge. Your feet sinking down slightly into the soft, warm ground. You lie facing the waterfall so you can enjoy this fairy spectacular until there is nothing left to watch. The warm earth caresses your side, your arm coming to rest under your head. You wonder if this is a birth of life, or simply a fresh start. These beings so graceful, and pure make no sound as they rise into the unknown.

Your eyes begin to feel heavy, so you rest them, for only a moment. It is now that you are starting to realize the power you have within you. Like these fairies you can sink down into this warm fresh start. Feel the bubble of your covers caressing you. Allowing you to relax and prepare for a new tomorrow.

This magical place is inside your mind, you have a gift unlike the other creatures before you. You can envision anything you want. There is a magical world in each of us, and it is different for everyone. It is perfect for everyone. Let it relax you, you have the power and the control to just let go.

Bedtime Stories for Adults

The Tranquil Submarine

You feel the breeze on your face, cool as is blows over the surreal blue ocean surrounding you. You are on your way to explore the magical world of the ocean by submarine. The excitement is coursing through your body, holding your muscles stiff. You have arrived at the submarine, you stand in line, awaiting to walk the stairs down through the port hole. It is finally your turn, as you descend the stairs you come into the submersible and feel your nerves ramp up a notch as your surroundings close in. Going from the vast ocean openness around you, down into a small vessel makes your body feel even more tense. You see the many windows lining the craft, with comfortable seating in front of each.

You eagerly make your way to your seat and sit down, allowing the plush comfort to cradle your body. Your body feels fidgety and antsy as you try to sink into the comfort, let's try to calm your nerves before this journey. Inhale deeply, allowing the oxygen to reach every organ in your body. Slowly exhale, relaxing the organs as they patiently await the next inhale. As people settle in around you, ignore them, focus only on yourself. Focus on this remarkable journey you're about to experience, seeing a new side of this precious gift of life from below the water's surface. Inhale in, allowing the cool breeze of

Lucy Holden

your breath travel through your body, down to toes and in between, caressing your feet, allowing them to relax as the breath warms and travels back, ready to be exhaled. Inhale again, this time focusing on the breath to travel down to your hands, in between your fingers, caressing your palms, as the breath warms and travels back to be exhaled. Inhale deeply, allowing the breath to settle your stomach, warming as it caresses your lungs, travels between your shoulder blades and back to exhale. Inhale deeply once more as the breath caresses your brain, warms it, comforts it, and then back to exhale.

You feel calm and relaxed as the pilot comes across the speaker to prepare you for descent. He tells you to pay close attention to the right side of the vessel as the submarine descends. You turn and see a family of sea lions. A slight shift in pressure reminds you that your body is snug inside this vessel, but let it be a snugness of comfort. The friendly and curious beings approach the vessel, delighting in the bubbles as you descend. Count to see how many sea lions there are. One, two, three, four, five, six, seven; there are seven playful sea lions. They swim quickly around the submarine. One swims up to your window, looking at you as you look at it. Its curious deep brown eyes filled with wonder and excitement, reflecting the wonder in your own. As the submarine continues to descend down the creatures lose interest and swim back to where they were.

Bedtime Stories for Adults

Staring out into the vast blueness of the ocean, you reflect on how hectic your life has become. How simple these creatures have it, just exist. Go through every day seeing the beauty in the world, living in it, enjoying it. You start to see small schools of fish, the pilot informs you of some of the species, but you drown out his talking a let it become a soft, lulling murmur in the background. You see fish that are bright blue with yellow tails. They dart this way and that way, minding their own business as the vessel passes them by. You see silver fish, some with stripes, some stream lined for speed, some with large graceful fins and a touch of color, traveling in the safety of numbers. All your thoughts from the day are clustered in packs like the fish in this ocean. A small shark soars by, some scatter away, some stick together and ignore the danger. Let's put those thoughts away, just let it be you here, nothing to distract your mind. Visualize the thoughts, now wrap them in a bubble and send them to the surface. They will be there for you on the surface, when you're ready for them. Each and every thought should be sent away in a bubble, watch the bubbles drift to the surface as you keep descending. Let them move further away from you, from your mind, until your mind is clear.

The pilot announces that we are off the coast of an island with lots of unusual creatures, you look closely out your window and see a lizard swim by. Unusual indeed. The

Lucy Holden

pilot tells you that these are marine iguanas and they are only in this area of the world. The small monster with deep green skin, with hints or red and orange, it is beautiful as it swims down onto the vivid green moss-covered rocks. You see a few more as you travel along.   Some resting on the colorful rocks, some chasing food, some swimming peacefully. The water is so clear and exquisite, it's like being in the world's largest aquarium from the inside. Seeing these creatures in their natural environment, seeing the wonder of their magnificent world is awe inspiring. You pass through a school of many slender fish, it seems there is more fish than water at this point. The fish are so thick the submarine gets briefly dark, it's just thousands and thousands of the narrow-bodied fish outside the windows.   Through the thickness, you see a bird glide through the water to snatch some of the fish for an easy meal. It is a penguin. Here in this tropical water, you see a penguin. You listen back in for the pilot to explain that these penguins are also indigenous to these islands. Who would have thought of all these wonderful creatures existing in this one magical place? You see another penguin dive down, do a spin, then dart back up. Its body streamlined for this job of hunting these particular fish.

You realize your body has become tense again as you've moved closer and closer to the window, afraid you will

Bedtime Stories for Adults

miss something. Sit back, relax, focus on your breathing and just enjoy what you can see. You will not miss anything. Out your window you can see a sting ray, almost black in color with white dots all over. The stingray gently lifts its wings revealing its white underside as it glides away from the vessel. As you move deeper away from the bright corals and rock and fish you notice the ocean is more open. Cold, and dark. You take the blanket off your chair and pull it snug around you. Blocking out the cold, but welcoming the dark as the low lights on the submarine flick on. The fish are more solitary now, hesitant of the vessel instead of curious. You see a large shark pass by, ignoring the submarine... the shark drifts by in its daily routine. There will be no more descending the pilot announces and you're grateful. You feel deep in the ocean, but the peace and quiet you're experiencing is unlike any other.

Out your window you see a sunken ship. It looks old, lonely, and desolate. But it is now also a haven for many fish away from the coral. You see smaller fish darting around the ship. The local life taking over what was once a part of your world. There is an odd sensation of peace, knowing that you are in their territory, these sharks, these fish, this deep, desolate ocean. This is their home, you are only here to visit, and they don't seem to mind. Some notice you, some don't even bother, they just let you admire. Admire how something old, tired, and broken can become something new and beautiful. This shipwreck is beautiful; harboring so much life around it. The lights illuminate how this ship belongs here now. These animals rely on its existence. This mistake that caused this ship to sink, was crucial to the survival of these animals here now. Everything is connected, everything happens for some reason. You may not always understand, but all you can do is relax and control how you feel. How your mind handles the things around you. You can have a peaceful and meaningful existence. Like this ship or like the animals around it. You have a purpose, and you will reach that purpose because that is life. The submarine travels on, leaving the ship behind.

As you leave everything behind your mind feels tired, the coldness of the ocean tries to sink through the walls of the vessel, but the cold doesn't touch you; the blanket is a warm comfort around you. You lie your head back and see through the top glass of the submarine. As your neck relaxes, like the rest of your body, you breath slowly as a huge sea turtle gracefully glides over the submarine. You can barely see the surface anymore, the dappled sunlight dancing faintly in the dark blue water. The turtle a dark silhouette, the occasional fish, big and small swimming above. Your body feels heavy, but relaxed. Your mind moving slow and peaceful as you take in the surroundings of the deep, vast ocean.   Close your eyes as you memorize the surroundings to hold with you forever. You will always recall this peace during times of stress, you will be able to close your eyes, seeing the ocean's surface way above you as the creatures' drift peacefully overhead.

Lucy Holden

The Dream Life

Just when you think life cannot get any worse than it currently is, either something magical can happen that will change your luck or it gets a little bit worse. Those are the only two options, after today you wonder how your luck will go, will it better? Or will your life come crashing down around you? You hear a knock on the door, your tired body drags you to answer it. You open the door to see a business woman, smiling largely as she hands you a heavy briefcase. Puzzled you don't want her to release the case. Who is this woman? Why is she here? Your brain struggles to process this, then she starts talking.

"You are the winner of the dream life sweepstake. You are the luckiest person on Earth right now, and everything is going to change for the better." This feels like a gimmick, surely, she will say you only need to invest, blah, blah, blah. So, you tell her that you are not interested and you just want her to leave you in peace so you can rest. She is dumfounded as you shut the door in her face.

As you walk back to your bed, your phone rings. You answer it to hear a formal voice on the other line announce that he's a lawyer for the World's richest man,

Bedtime Stories for Adults

a man who died a few weeks ago. In his will he had a list of names, people that he had encountered in his life...everyone from the school librarian in primary school to a drive thru window cashier at the McDonald's. Anyone he met, he added them to this list. Upon his death he wanted his list to become a sweepstakes for his fortune, but his money ruined his life. It tore apart his family, it made him greedy, it made him lazy. He wants someone to be able to live out their dream life, through his will, but with guidance. The lady at the door is the first step towards guiding you to accepting this fortune. After the lawyer explains, you still can't seem to process this. You don't think you met this man, and if you had...would you be so lucky as to win his entire fortune?

Is this that point where your luck changes? Will it be the best thing that ever happened to you? Or will you waste your time? Isn't it worth the amount of time, just to listen to the lady? What harm can it do? You turn around and walk back to the door. Allowing the woman to enter your home. You have a seat at the table and she opens the brief case. "First, we will start with a questionnaire. I am to guide you to a dream life, not just hand you a fortune. Once that I am certain you are ready to have the fortune, it will be all yours." You hesitantly agree, still feeling this is too good to be true.

Lucy Holden

What is your dream job, do you wish to earn fulfillment through your work, or is it a means to an end? You decide you have nothing to hide from this woman, so you tell her the truth. She nods and moves on to the next question.

What is your dream family? Do you have it? Would money change your family, for the better or for the worse?

If you could live anywhere in the world, where would you live? Why would you live there?

"Ok, that takes care of the basics. Give me a few moments and I'll be back soon." As she leaves the room, you suddenly find yourself a bundle of nerves. Your body is tense and achy. You want to relax yourself, not let this work you up. So, you take a deep breath in as you stretch and flex the muscles in your body. As you exhale slowly, you allow the muscles to relax. You can feel a warm tingling sensation rushing through as you repeat the process. You keep breathing in slowly, becoming aware of your body. It is heavy and tired, you relax into the chair and focus on the simple task of breathing and allowing your body to rest. The lady enters the room again and you feel relaxed, maybe this is for the best. "Now, we will start building your dream life. Starting with some major purchases, then working through the minor ones so we can organize your new life. What type of car do you wish to have? Do you need anything custom on it?" She hands you a form, as you order your dream car.

You think about all the cars you've wanted throughout your life, until you finally settle on one. You try to keep in mind, this is because you're not spending your own money. This is just a 'dream' car for a reason.   Think of every elaborate detail you would want in that car, including a personal driver, if that's what you want. Once you have etched every detail into that paper, hand it back to her.

"Now, we can decide on your land. I got some listings in the areas you described as your dream location. Please, look over these and see if any of them are what you had in mind."

As you look through the real estate listings, you see so many perfect opportunities. They are exactly where you would want to build a dream home. You look at the surrounding areas and you can picture the beautiful landscape now. Hearing the local noises. Smelling the scents, feeling the peace it would bring to you to be there now. You realize you've held onto this particular listing for a while. You let her know this is the one you like the most. Her fingers fly across her phone as she informs you that the land now belongs to you. All the paperwork will be signed at the end. You are dumbfounded as you look at her and ask, "Why me? How did I know this man, why would he want to give me this dream life?"

"I don't know the details. I just know that your name was on his list, and it is the name that was selected. My job is planned out in exquisite details, which is why we are able to shuffle along through these tasks. You are in fact a very lucky person, with a great fortune. Let's not lose momentum now, the sooner we have everything in order, the sooner you get to experience your dream life. The best contractor and his team are prepared to draw up your dream house when you are ready. They will be here shortly, I have just sent them the land, so they will have a better idea on how to make things work for you. While we wait for them, are you happy in your current dwellings? Or do you want a new temporary home while your dream home is being constructed?"

You think long and hard on the question. Now that money is apparently not a problem, what do you want to do while your dream home is being constructed? Do you want to live here and just wait? Do you want to hire movers and move into a nice upscale place? Or a place far away from everyone and everything while you process your new life? Surely, you'll want to escape the media, if you stay in your current dwellings, you need people to help keep the media off you. Or maybe you'll step into the spot light and shine, embracing your dream life. When you thought of what you wanted you let the lady know and she assures you that nothing will be a problem. All your wishes for your new life will be answered.

The contractor has arrived with his team, only now that it is not just this lady in front of you, or the voice on the phone from earlier, the reality is really sinking in. Your life is going to become everything you've ever wanted. As they bring in their things and get settled you start to wonder what you will do with your life? With all your worries fading quicker and quicker into your past, what does your soul want? When everything material in this world becomes easily bought, what are the things you need to work on? How can you be the person that you truly want to be? Do you need all this money to accomplish your goals? Will it make your life that much easier? Probably, but when all those little inconveniences are covered, and no longer troublesome, does your life feel empty or is there a vast opening that you can now explore? Will you travel the world? Will you fund new charities or help those already established?

The contractor introduces himself and starts to ask questions about your dream home so that they may begin the process...you feel your mind flood with images of beautiful houses, but you don't know where to start. You inhale and exhale and decide right now to start becoming the new you, as you describe this home. This home reflects who you are as a person. Build it from the ground up. Describe how you want your base, in detail, build your dream home, until you drift into a deep peaceful rest. When you wake up tomorrow, you will be this new person with a strong base to work on your dream life.

The Ocean's Song

You are on a small, remote island. The sand and ocean pristine, the vegetation is full and lively. Simple living is a way of life here and it feels like time itself passes slower. There is no hurrying about as you decide to go for a walk on the remarkable beach. The sun is low in the sky, the air is warm and perfect. The glistening sand is soft, almost white in color as your feet sink slowly and softly into the warm, welcoming sand with each step. Allowing the warmth to spread around your feet, but not stick as you gracefully stroll along the water's edge. The water to your right is a beautiful Caribbean blue, with white foam bubbles as the waves gently caress the beach.

As you slowly walk you can hear the ocean; seeming to swell in the great distance, but when it reaches you it is a

Bedtime Stories for Adults

soft whisper. A remnant of the great wave it once was. If the ocean were a person, what things could it tell you? Would it tell you of its survival? Of its suffering? Of the astounding life it provides for many? Would it sing it in a song? Listen to the ocean. Can you hear it sing? Is it a sweet lullaby? Is it singing ever so softly? As you watch the waves dancing to the song you yearn to feel them caress your skin.   Walking just barely into the water, feel the waves crash upon your tired feet.

Feel the sand beneath you give way as the earth pulls you down. Stand still, allow the ocean to embrace you. The coolness of the water quickly passes as the next wave surrounds your ankles. Allowing your feet to sink just a little further into the warm sand. As the water sways out you feel your body call out to it to come back. It does, it always does. The water goes out, it comes back in. The ocean breathes, just like you. The water comes in, you take a deep breath, filling your lungs with oxygen. You breath out, the water rushes out. Carrying that sweet oxygen from your head down to your emerged toes. Listen to the ocean's song as it breaths with you. Swaying with the gentle sounds, settling your body down into the earth. Like the roots of a tree, you are beneath the earth now while still reaching for the sky. Anchored into the life-giving solid base of this planet.

Lucy Holden

You hear a giggle in the distance, instantly recognizing the tinkling sound; as a young child plays on the beach. Such pure joy and happiness pull you towards it. As you approach the child you give a warm welcome. They giggle and continue in their own little world of happiness. Slightly ahead there is a bench. You decide to sit for a while and just enjoy the scenery. The sun low over the ocean, the palm trees behind you swaying with the light breeze. The sand soft and warm, glistening the reflection of the sun. You lie your head back allowing your neck to relax as you listen to the sounds. The ocean singing its song as it breathes in and out. The child's soft giggles of pure joy and happiness. This place is paradise, it is as if there is no room for the cloudy thoughts of tomorrow. For the doubts in the recesses of your mind. All your troubles need to escape.

You feel a soft tap on your shoulder and you open your eyes to see the sweet child smiling at you. The child hands you a container of bubbles. Without speaking any words, you know this child is asking you to blow the bubbles for them. You feel silly, playing with this child, but there is no harm. You open the bubbles, dip the wand, and exhale gently. A stream of iridescent bubbles spews forth. The child giggles and dances as they fall around them. You feel yourself smile, knowing the very simple effort you put forth caused someone else such great joy is a rewarding sensation. You repeat a few

Bedtime Stories for Adults

times, but the child's parent is calling for them. They run off abruptly, you try to call them back, hand them the bubbles, but they are gone.

Left alone with your thoughts and the child's play you speak to your inner child. What do you want in life? You ask it. As your mind responds, you blow a big, soft bubble and watch it drift off. Your mind is settled making the exchange, a bubble is just as good as an answer on this island. Anything that is on your mind, form it into the bubble. Blow it away. No matter how big or small, each bubble is satisfying to just let go. Collect each and every though you have, pouring them into this bubble liquid. Dip in the wand, and blow them all away. This is your time for relaxation. Nothing stands in your way except your mind. Who controls your mind? Control each thought as you form consistent beautiful bubbles. Watch them drift over the ocean. Carrying your troubles away from you.

Watching the bubbles disappear over the ocean you notice the sun is now even lower in the sky. There is still no rush. Nothing to hurry to, nothing to worry you; simply be and enjoy. The sun is wrapped in magical, striking colors. Above the sky is pink, turning to a warm orange and yellow glow surrounding the sun. The clouds white up high and sinking down to grey, to darkest of blue just above the ocean. The purple just above the horizon starts so soft near the sun and sinks down into the black of night. You can see the stars starting to wake up throughout the sky. Twinkling to life as the day shifts into the night.

With the darkness settling in you decide to make your way to your island retreat. The sand is different now. No longer warm as your feet sink into the calm coolness of the sand is still welcoming. One thing that is consistent is the song of the ocean. Although it is no longer a whisper, it sings louder, encouraging you to experience the steady cadence. Breathing in, breathing out as you meander your way to your home away from home. You can see the soft glow of the porch light, but you also see the shadow of the hammock in the side yard. The hammock calls to you, you aren't ready to turn off the ocean's song just yet.

Nestled between two great palm trees, you climb into hammock. As you sway, you find your center of balance. Focusing your breathing with the faint song of the ocean. Breathing gently in, you allow your feet to rest. Breathing out you allow your legs to sink into the sturdy net beneath you. Breathing in, your back and stomach settle and as you breath out they sigh into the perfect position of comfort. Resting your arms comfortably you allow the breath to continue influencing your relaxation. The frogs and insects start to come alive and sing their own songs. They do not distract you; your song has become your own reflexive action. Breathing in and breathing out is the natural order. You no longer need to think of actively doing it, your body will just continue to do this as your muscles stay relaxed and your bones settled.

You peer up through the outline of the huge palm fronds and see every star in the night sky. The moon is a tiny sliver, as if handing over the spotlight of the night sky to the stars. Allowing them to share their beauty with you. You begin to draw patterns and shapes between the stars. Do you see the bear? The man with his bow and arrows? The queen sitting upon her throne? The swan, flying gracefully through the night? Tracing the connections between each group. Do you just see many lines, connecting all the stars? Focus harder, look at each individual star.

Imagine how much life and potential there is that is seeing this same star as you at this very moment. In the big scheme you are no different than any other, yet you are a thousand ways unique. You have so much inside you, but you are in control of it all. Every thought you have, is a part of you. You control where that thought is stored. If it's troublesome, blow it away in a bubble. If it is pleasant, explore it. This is your time, your vacation, you are everything in existence and you are nothing but quiet and stillness. Allow your eyes to rest like the rest of your body. Let them be sleepy and at peace. Give your mind control of your entire body; your mind gives you peace, joy, and rejuvenation. Nourish it, enjoy the song of your mind as you drift into oblivion.

The Changing Seasons

The seasons, they change. It is not sad, happy, or with frustration, it just simply is. Just like the seasons change, so do we. Do you let your seasons simply change as you move through life, or do you try to force them to stay the same or force them to move on too soon? Just like the rotation of the Earth, there are some things in this life you cannot control. These are things we need to learn to accept as graciously as possible. It is not always easy, but with practice and knowledge, just like everything else in life; we learn to deal with our seasons changing. You can think of your season as a day in your life, or maybe a time period. However large scale or small scale you need to picture the answer is what feels right for you, what brings you the most peace.

Picture you are a great big oak tree. As you stretch your body tall, your roots have grown deep down into the earth. The rains you have felt, have made you dig down deeper, sturdy your foundation. Your bark is tired as it keeps your body rigid. The early spring wind blows through, making you sway a little as you creak and sigh. Think of your bark as your blanket, pull it close to you, let it surround you in its warmth as it supports your growth. Let this growth warm you from the inside out. Focusing your breathing as it spreads from deep down

Lucy Holden

on the tips of your roots, all the way up to new leaves blossoming to life. As you feel the sun warming you up from the outside, you are now completely surrounded in warmth.   The sun is essential for your growth, feeding you joy and happiness. Your branches spreading out and settling into their new relaxing fullness as your thoughts in your busy mind appear as leaves upon your branches. Your leaves filling out with new green as all the thoughts fill every single leaf. This may be your early life, from the time you were a child, growing into a young adult. Each leaf holding new meaning, new thoughts, new memories, anything that rests within your mind can be found on a new green leaf. As you picture each thought in your mind, blossom it into a leaf. This can be any thoughts you have, maybe from your early, or maybe just from today. Once your tree is full of new green thought leaves, so full it cannot hold anymore, it is time for the day to change.

As the days begin to grow longer, the sun warmer. Let your thoughts begin to settle. As each thought becomes full, it grows into a deep summer green. Some thoughts are fleeting in your summer days, maybe you enrich the lives of the insects as they rest and sing you beautiful songs in return for some nourishment from your thoughts. It's ok to let go of these leaves, let the insects take them. Maybe a summer thunderstorm passes through. The rains and wind taking away your thought leaves before they're ready to go on their own. This is natural, summer is an enriching time in our lives, but it can also be unpredictable. During summer there is growth, mature growth. Growth from being a young adult, to an adult. Growth from being too busy to experience life to knowing there are things in life you should slow down to enjoy. Summer can be warm and pleasant, or it can be sweltering and nearly unbearable. You are a full, deep green oak tree. You are tired and your leaves rest heavy on you, the summer days are almost over and you can feel the air calling out for you to take a rest.

Maybe Summer for you is going from a young adult to an adult. Maybe it was the rough part of the day that is time to just let go of. Just as the seasons will surely change, so will your life, so will your day.

The air becomes crisp, your senses sharpened with wisdom. You know the joy of growth has come and is nearly time for its end. You feel the deep green thoughts begin to change. What had once felt urgent and important fade to wonderful and colorful shades of yellow, orange, and red. The change being so visible, you know it is nearly time to let them go. As the smallest rustle or whisper of wind causes those thoughts that are too full to drift slowly to the ground. Let them go, they are no longer part of what you need. What your mind needs now is relaxation and wonderful peace. It is

Lucy Holden

Autumn, it is Fall, it is time to let go. Watch in wonder as your thoughts become less meaningful, less impactful on your life as they drift slowly to the ground. Surrounding you in a colorful blanket.

Maybe Autumn for you is going from an adult to accepting the wisdom and maturity that come with age. To embracing that age with pride, knowing that it is just a season you must go through. Maybe it is acceptance for the things you cannot change, but embracing the wisdom that you get from experiencing the many trials and tribulations throughout life. Or is it just the part of the day where you can slow down, breath, and start to relax. Isn't it peaceful knowing that all the growth, and business of the day is finally over... you can let the responsibilities drift away like the leaves surrounding you.

You feel a change in the air around you, the coolness begins to become frigid. This is your mind reminding you of all the leaves you have lost. This is the harshness of Winter. This is the hardest season to control or predict and this is what you experience at the end of each cycle of seasons. Whether it is the end of your day, or towards the end of your life. Maybe you have a short winter and the frigid night passes quickly. Or maybe you are packed up tight and you're prepared for the harshness of winter. I am here to help you deal with your Winter. Remember that you are a strong oak tree, with a thick, warm blanket of bark to protect you. Your leaf thoughts have gone and left you bare to the dark and cold of night. How do you get through this desolate loneliness? Just your body and your empty mind. For starters you are not alone. You are the greatest company that you will ever know. You know yourself better than anyone. You know what you want from life. Your mind knows how to get it, even if you're unsure, deep down you know you will figure it out. Stop thinking of Winter as the end of the cycle. It is your new beginning, a chance to start over. It is the peaceful calm where you know you must rest; before the life of Spring wakes up. During Winter, you don't worry about what Spring will hold. Just allow the Winter to surround you, live in it.

Allow the snow to fall, surround you. It is not cold, but it is heavy. Let its weight be a comfort as it forces your muscles and your body to stay relaxed. If you feel tense, the heavier the blanket of snow will become, until you have finally given over to the relaxation. Allow your mind to welcome the white, peaceful new blanket surrounding it. Your day is over, there is no reason to think of it any longer. It is not yet time for Spring, so do not think of tomorrow. Let this be your day to enjoy Winter. Live in the state of rest.

Lucy Holden

Maybe Winter for you is the final stage of life. A time where you have no more worries. You are retired, your family is settled and happy. You have come to accept that life has been through most of its highs and it is time to just rest. Enjoy being in complete calm, nothing is expected, nothing is anticipated. Maybe Winter is the end of the day. The time at night when your mind has gracefully decided to let go of the day's thoughts. To let you drift off to sleep with no expectations. Just calm and blissful sleep to rejuvenate your mind, your daily Winter. This rest is needed, so that your mind can prepare itself for the busy Spring ahead. This is the season that we all try to skip over, because we feel it isn't vital for growth.

One can argue that it is the most vital, because without this period of rest; the more ragged we become. The harder our other seasons seem. As the seasons change, so must we. We need to be able to set aside the time of our days to transition smoothly. When it is time to let go, let the season change. Embrace the end of the cycle, rest in your Winter before you move on.